Igniting your Weight Loss Motivation

Five proven steps to get you back on track!

Achievement Pyramid

Table of Contents

Introduction

I want to thank you and congratulate you for downloading the book, ***"Igniting your weight loss motivation"***.

This book contains proven steps and strategies on how to rekindle the needed fire to get you motivated to work on your body and lose weight.

This book presents a unique opportunity for those who find it difficult to do the needful, those who have tried and failed to start and maintain a weight loss program, a dietary program or the regular visits to the gym. This book will clearly show you a few proven steps that should help you get back on track if you were ever on one or to help you discover the right track at weight loss if you have never discovered one.

Thanks again for downloading this book, I hope you enjoy it!

reader. Under no circumstances will any legal responsibility or blame be held against the publisher for any reparation, damages, or monetary loss due to the information herein, either directly or indirectly.

Respective authors own all copyrights not held by the publisher.

The information herein is offered for informational purposes solely and is universal as so. The presentation of the information is without a contract or any type of guarantee assurance.

The trademarks that are used are without any consent, and the publication of the trademark is without permission or backing by the trademark owner. All trademarks and brands within this book are for clarifying purposes only and are the owned by the owners themselves, not affiliated with this document.

Chapter 1 :Getting Motivated

Motivation is basically everything! From getting your home properly cleaned to maintaining a particular diet, motivation gives you the required will power that backs up your every step and also helps you achieve every one of your desires.

If your motivation is at a crescendo, you are bound to feel quite energized, determined, focused and driven. Nothing is going to be able to stop a motivated man even if it means doing stuff that he is not cool with. You simply get to work, cleaning your home, sending the letter and getting started on that diet. Not one of these appears like a challenge, you simply get to it right? Well, this all go?

However at some point, something creeps into your life and appears to deflate you of all the motivation. It could be a challenge with your health, a family challenge. It could be a change of environment as well, change of employment, a breakup. Soon, you lose focus and you appear to lack motivation and before long you are back to square one. The things that you had under control soon get back to where they were before. The dirty clothes pile up in the house, you seem to gain even more weight and your frequent visit to the gym becomes an occasional event.

Remaining motivated doesn't necessarily mean that you must remain excited and strong every single day. However, you only need to know how to get yourself back on your feet when the need arises. For someone who wants to achieve a goal, motivation is what makes you stay focused and consistent with whatever plan such as exercise plans. Motivation is what makes you wake up early in the day and go on long walks and runs. Motivation is what makes you keep at it in the cold, pressures notwithstanding. Nothing should be able to stop a motivated man from carrying out his daily routine.

However, a motivated person passes through times when things happen which tends to make them lose steam. When this occurs, it is only smart that you come up with a plan to overcome the struggle that takes place on Sunday night and the reality of Monday morning. One person described this by saying that she feels quite motivated just the night before.

However, when morning comes and the alarm rings and it's just 4:30 am and she still feels like she has the whole world loaded on her body. She says that she speaks positive words to herself and reminds herself of the rewards. However, in her words "nothing seems to get those sheets off my body, soon I turn off the annoying alarm and change gear for a better sleeping experience for about an hour or so more."

The simple fact is that motivation requires some bit of energy. Whenever you feel like you have lost steam, stressed, or overwhelmed, there is every chance that you will find it difficult to keep on moving. Despite the fact that you must be aware that exercise should get your looking and feeling much better, you just cannot get yourself to get it done. Between settling on the sofa with a cheese burger and going out for a walk, the sofa always wins.

It is vital to recognize that staying motivated is a product of a conscious decision, however, motivation does not just fall down from heaven or evaporate after a while. You can't open your bag and be like, "hey! I've found my motivation!" however, your energy and drive which ensures that you are on the right track come from within. Even though it seems like it just comes unannounced, it is actually a product of choice. It is of your own making via yourself speeches, your disposition as well as the thoughts of your heart.

Due to the fact that the energy and drive come from your heart, you certainly have all it takes to get yourself motivated whenever the need arises. Even when you feel totally weak, you should still be able to get motivated if you really want to. Instead of tarrying for inspiration to come, you should definitely learn how you can bring it out yourself. In order to get this done, you ought to be able to come up with new ideas and tricks which should get you motivated towards the goal. However, at some stage, you will need to get up from your comfort zone and ensure that it happens

Chapter 2 :Waking up the Motivation

Here, you will learn some steps that should help you wake up the motivation when it appears to fade off. Although there are a few of them outline, you may need to place focus on one of them per time, getting to work on each one until you have triumphed in that particular area.

 However, you may opt to address the five concepts all at the same time and make use of them to kick-start your actions and get yourself back in line. Whichever way, you will certainly be surprised as to how effective these steps are once you begin to implement them. Aside from helping you to get your motivation back for the mean time; they should also get you the right plan for attaining success in the long run.

First step

Conquer and divide

At Mary's weight loss program, people participating will always come up with a weekly goal for the week to come. However, Mary decided against to engage in this segment. In her words, "I dislike exercises and I am just not wanted to engage in It." Other members of the group backed up her decision and enjoined her to ensure she keeps on attending the group notwithstanding.

Hence, every other week, she came to the meetings however, she decided against writing out a list of goals. However, one day, she spoke up subtly "I have a bike at the back of my room, maybe I might just begin making use of it time after time". Soon after saying this everyone appeared to try to help her with the plan, "awesome plan Mary! Try it out; just ensure you begin small so that you do not become tired of it." Hence, Mary listed on a sheet, "I will use my bike each day for two minutes," the week after, the members of the group were eager to hear of her progress. "I succeeded! " She exclaimed "each day is used my bike for two minutes. I am sure of this because I made use of my watch."

The week that followed, Mary reported on her success yet again. However, at this point, she agreed to up her aim for 5 minutes each day. Again, she recorded success. As time went by, Mary began increasing in progress from five minutes to 30 minutes each day.

One year after, Mary who found it hard to exercise had lost about 50 pounds by running five miles each and every day. In Mary's words "the thought of exercise overwhelmed me so much that I couldn't event begin. Setting little goals was all it took to start on the road to success."

Get it broken up

When you get to work on a something different, ensure that you break up your goals into fragmented goals, instead of addressing it all at the same time. Nicole was quite discouraged about her chances of shedding about 170 pounds. Hence, she made a choice to focus on her dietary program until she had lost about 30 pounds, after which she carried out a re-evaluation of her objectives.

When she attained her initial focus, she considered her efforts rather carefully and then made a decision to shed another 30 pounds. Sherry engaged in this system for about five times during the course of her program, each time carrying out a re-evaluation of her plans at the conclusion of each one of the 30-pounds loss. At the start, she couldn't see herself attaining her weight-loss goals; however, by the end of the year, she had lost about 150 pounds

15-Pound Goals

You should also be able to attain and manage your weight loss projections by simply setting small targets such as losing 15 pounds. This is how Paul came over his discouragement as regards the number of pounds he needed to shed. When his weight was still within the range of 290 pounds, Paul coined a phrase that has helped him in maintaining focus on his goals.

He simply told himself, "You will not be able to get to 220 except to attain 275." Thereafter, he placed great emphasis on shedding the next 15 pounds. Every single time he attained his 15-pounds goal, he would simply modify the numbers in his statement. This is what made a big change in his thoughts and disposition, it also helped in no great measure attain his desired weight of 220 pounds.

Chapter 3 :Make your Intentions known

The summer before now, Lisa got herself a brand new diet book. The book contained plans that could only be described as awesome and Lisa was aware of the fact that if she actually followed the plans religiously, chances were high that should would shed about 40 pounds quite easily.

However, it soon turned out to be that this was a little complex hence she soon has some challenge knowing what exactly it is she was supposed to eat. Whenever she made up her mind to adhere to the diet plan, the right type of food was or the needed time to religiously follow the plan.

Lisa was really bent on making it work, hence she stuck to her inner belief that someday she would carve out time to take a good look at the book and make use of the plan contained therein. One year on, and Lisa has not yet begun the diet. The sad part of it is that she still weighs as much as she did the year before, however, she feels a lot more disgusted and frustrated about herself.

Get the Motivation revived

Motivation requires an end result just like Lisa, Perhaps; you have had it at the back of your mind to begin a diet or create a plan for exercise, but never began. First came the graduation, the vacations as well as weddings. Then it got to a point where it got virtually impossible to picture planning and cooking. Sooner rather than later, it would be fall season and that means your chances of fitting into the summer bikini would all but evaporate.

Vague thoughts such as "I desire to lose some weight" never really give you the needed resolve. However, when you set for yourself exercise and weight-loss goals, ensure that you measurable results. For instance, you may set for yourself goals like "I desire to weight about 150 pounds by the month of September" or "I desire to run a run a 4 mile without needing to reduce my pace." Setting specific targets would certainly help you get better motivated than when you when you just say "let me try this and see what comes out of it."

Maintain or lose weight?

Are you the type of individual who always says " I have a great desire to shed weigh" but never act on it? Except you have plans to add more weight, you basically have just two options-to maintain or lose your current weight. However, ensure you don't say one thing and do something different.

If you really desire really want to lose the pounds and then face it squarely. Be particular about your exercise and diet plan, then think of a way to make it work out. Keep count of your points or calories. Take rides on your bike, go on long walks or go to the local gym and shed some weight. What this means is that, ensure you execute your intents. Regardless of your intent at losing some weight, the goal may not appear to be feasible.

There is absolutely nothing wrong as regards shedding weight-however, ensure that it's your target and live by it. If not, you will just remain frustrated due to the fact that your mind says a thing but the things you do say something different.

Indecision is a big decision

If you are unable to make a decision as regards your being willing to adhere to a particular exercise or a diet, then you should know you are in trouble. The simple truth is that your inability to arrive at a decision is basically a decision in its self. Without having a clear-cut plan, you will definitely end up doing just about nothing in particular.

You could basically end up wasting a whole lot of your energy and time telling yourself "I will begin soon". Hence, except you are ready to make a step, don't ever say those words, and be sincere with yourself. If you are not yet totally ready to shed some weight now, then stop feeling guilty and just tarry until the time is right. Instead, invest your energy into keeping your weight maintained.

Chapter 4 :Becoming unstuck

Lois was stuck! She had been a manager at a big company for about 12 years. She had it all, a great job, cool income, however, the stress and politics that played out in her department were giving her a really tough time. In one of the coaching visitations, she lamented how she was feeling unhappy at work; however, she could not get to the point where she would change her job.

On a good day, she gave a graphic description of just how trapped she really was, she was given a piece of paper which had the following words written on it: for how long do I intend living like this? She was challenged to give a response to the question the next week. Her response was to be specific, like deciding to leave things the way they were for half a year or even a year.

Joan went home with the paper and had it glued to her refrigerator. Later that day, she opened it and read it while she continued thinking about the different times she could give a response. Suddenly she realized, she really did not want to stay in that same situation, not even for one extra minute. The next day, Lois resigned from her work.

Once Lois took that step, she soon discovered that the other changes just about came easily. For about half a year, she began operating a consulting company, she also lost about sixty pounds and she put in for the Peace Corps.

 What's more? She soon became an addicted exerciser, going on her bike to her new office. At about 50 years of age, just 3 years after she left her "depressing job", she got her first assignment with the Peace Corps and she soon began going all over the world. Lois is in no way stuck! She said, "When I discovered I had no intention of living that way again, it basically became the drive I needed to effect changes in some other dysfunctional areas of my life."

Are you feeling awful like Lois, when you are not feeling motivated, there is always a chance that you would get stuck and thus become hopeless about things ever becoming better? Perhaps you keep telling yourself that you will change, but you just never bring yourself to act on it. When you get stuck, everything basically stops.

You might even desire some form of crisis due to the fact that you are certain that it's the only thing that keeps you moving. One thing you must understand about being stuck is that it assumes an identity in its self. Hence, instead of you working on the challenge, you keep pointing fingers at others for the steps you are not taking. However, if someone gives you any counsel, you get offended and say "you just don't know what I am going through"

The Deeper stuck

The simple reality of life is that everyone gets stuck at one point or the other, this is especially so when it has to do with losing weight or engaging in regular exercise. However, chances are high that you could get into a rut at your work, in your marriage, in a relationship and so on.

The fact is that as you get depressed or discouraged due to the fact that nothing seems to change, the rut simply gets deeper and deeper. At the end of the day, you just cannot see an escape route out of your frustrating life. You begin to have the belief that you have no other alternative and that there is nothing that can surmount your present predicament.

You simply stay the way you are instead of taking risks or attempting something new. People who get stuck usually remain that way for quite some time. By clinging to their rather skewed beliefs and attitudes, they go on building their lack of motivation. Before you can be able to escape the trap, you will have to face the reasons that are keeping you in that position.

Don't lose sight of the possibilities

Being stuck can compare to putting on opaque glasses when you take a look at the world. As far as life is concerned, it's quite easy to remain hung up on little challenges and lose focus on the other possible ways of getting things done. As a result of the fact that you cannot see the possibilities, you soon conclude that there is none.

I advise you to part with your beliefs that appear to limit you and instead take a look at the different new possibilities and check out the different other ways you can have things approached. This is a simple example of how it all works. Brenda had set for herself a goal of engaging in constant exercise for at least 6 days each week, however, each day, she found herself skipping her exercise while engaging in another exercise during the time frame. When she discovered that her motivation had all but gone away, she decided to come up with a list of things that could help her attain success.

Take note how creative she became the list increased.

Things that will drive me to exercise each day

- Ensure the alarm is set at least an hour earlier
- Spread out the exercise clothes before I sleep
- Fill the water bottle and put it in the refrigerator
- Make use of self-talk as soon as I wake
- Ensure that my tires are in good shape before I go to bed
- Go on my bike for only 7 blocks the first time
- Register with the nearby health club
- Engage a personal trainer
- Get new songs to hear while at it

It's now your own turn. Get a paper or simply turn on your PC and create a new document. Make a choice of the area that you desire to see changes and come up with a list of possible actions regardless of how small that should help you make meaningful progress. Carry this out with a number of goals such as maintaining a meal plan or including exercise in your daily routine. You can allow your imagination to do the rest of the job.

You will be surprised as to the number of options you will be able to come up with. When you open up your mind to new possibilities, you soon discover diverse ways to attain your aim. Instead of becoming hung up by the little obstacles in your life, have a great focus on the larger picture which brings fresh and unlimited possibilities

Chapter 5 :Increase Its Importance

It is quite interesting the way we tend to act in a different manner when we tag things as important. For example, if you view your final exam as vital, chances are high that you will stay awake till late, reject invites to parties and compel yourself to study.

When you really have a desire to get something, generating the needed motivation becomes quite easy. All you need to do is to increase the level of importance of the goal by raising it higher in terms of your priorities

It Matters if you make it a matter

Cherry had always had a desire to lose weight for quite a long period of time. Recently she had been a little bit more desperate; however, she was still having difficulties maintaining her diet plans. When she thought about the diverse ways through which her weight had negatively affected her life, she developed a rather long list.

How my weight has been affecting me

- ➢ I constantly feel miserable
- ➢ I have worries about my health
- ➢ My legs and feet always ache
- ➢ I find it difficult to put on really nice clothes
- ➢ It's really difficult to engage in exercise
- ➢ I look for reasons not to go out in public
- ➢ The seats at the theatre are no longer comfortable
- ➢ I worry too much about my looks
- ➢ I have low self-esteem

When Cherry assessed her condition, she told herself "when I take a look at this list, I know that my weight has a great effect on me. Almost every other day, I feel a lot miserable, I develop a hate for myself and I just wish that everything else was different."

As she began considering just how being overweight appeared to be disrupting her life, she concluded it was just about time to get to work. The day after, she made use of her newly discovered motivation to start a healthy exercise and dietary plan. Does this have any impact on you? Then you should start also.

Select one part of your life where you are struggling to be motivated. Aside from the issue of losing weight, you may also consider areas such as stopping smoking, quitting drinking, eating impulsively and exercising. Picture the diverse ways this areas of challenge affect your life as an individual. Does it impact your energy or your health? Is it negatively impacting your self-esteem does it make somehow challenging to manage your stress levels or emotions?

Making use of Cherry's work as an instance, come up with a list of different ways the challenge affects you in your life. Don't withhold anything. Write down every single thing that comes to your mind such as the number of gowns in your closet that no longer fits, the way the kids act embarrassed when they are with you in public. Make use of this list to drive you higher in terms of motivation, you can also make use of it to set for yourself goals aimed at removing the things you have noted down.

Create new reasons

When something does not really have much of an impact on your life, it is always quite difficult to generate the required motivation to effect a change.

One other way you could increase your motivation is to up the level of importance of your goals. So that it would matter even more. Take another deep look at how your weight, as well as other related and unrelated issues, affect you generally and if possible, come up with additional concerns.

Despite the fact that she had a desire to shed 30 pounds, Mary never really stayed on her diet for a long time enough to make any meaningful progress. However, aside from finding it quite difficult to fit into her business suits, she really didn't see any other reason why she should effect changes to her pattern. Mary excelled at her job, her health definitely was not an issue of concern, and most days she was totally oblivious to her weight.

Owing to the fact that it really didn't have much of an effect on her life, she found it quite difficult remaining motivated to do something about her added weight. However, when she took a closer look at her condition, she soon discovered some things that made her bothered aside her not being able to fit into her suits.

Mary's new list of why she should lose weight

> ➢ Be more comfortable putting on a bathing suit

> ➢ Develop greater self-confidence when in public
> ➢ Feel better when I look at myself in my mirror
> ➢ I want to begin a running program
> ➢ I want to attain a healthy weight before I get pregnant

By coming up with a few more reasons why she should lose her weight, Mary was able to up her motivation to a whole new level. This change was all she needed to start working on losing weight again. What do you really think you are willing to do? Once you have established how much such goals have an effect on your life, picture your reasons for being motivated to achieve it.

If you are the type that really does not care that much, you may have a number of days when you will not feel like being driven and you may just let things go the way they want to.

However, if you make a decision to do anything required, you will certainly improve your motivation. Hence, first and foremost, look out for ways through which your weight or any other issue may be having an effect on you as a person and create a deeper desire to have it changed.

Leverage on your support systems, self-talks as well as any other way you can work on your resolve as a person. Whenever your motivation goes south, take a journey back to your list and remind yourself of the fact that you are more than willing to act on getting yourself back on the right track.

CHAPTER 6 : Ignite your own fire

You have come up with your own goals and developed and action plan in that regard. Each and every day, you feel quite sure that you will begin your exercise or dietary plans. However, nothing appears to happen. The days go by and you have still not done anything. So how exactly do you ignite the fire which should help you in reviving your inner energy and get you on track yet again? The steps outlined in this final part are definitely sure to help you get yourself motivated while maintaining same motivation.

Just get something done!

Do you remember the first time you made a jump into the pool? Chances are high that you just stood on the bank of the pool waiting for long hours. Perhaps those guys behind you kept on telling you to hurry up, however, for some reason, you just could not move. When you finally got every single ounce of determination you could get, you made the jump. After you did it the first time, chances are high that you went right back to do it again. Surely it must have felt easier than the first time. However, for you to have made that first jump, you had to first break the barrier that was the first jump.

The simple truth is that sometimes, you just only need to take just a step and jump into the water. For instance, if you eat one healthy meal or take one walk, you should know that you have overcome the state of lack of motivation. Once you have begun, you will discover that it only gets easier to stay on in your program and maintain progress.

Every single time you lose motivation and struggle to get back on the right track, remind yourself of this phrase: just get something done, and then you have begun! Allow this concept to work for you repeatedly.

Even doing little things helps you become motivated as it helps you in breaking inertia and also helps to remind you of your internal power. Hence, take one bold step and overcome the rut and you will surely find yourself back in the mix.

The "Fifteen-Minute Solution"

When you find yourself in a situation where you just can't seem to get the needed motivation to begin exercising, make use of this idea to start off your efforts. Remind yourself that you only have to do it for 15 minutes, then you can throw in the towel.

After doing this, just get yourself through the door and go for a ride on your bike, take a walk or go to the local gym. You will be surprised as to how easy it is to get yourself moving. Knowing that you only need to do it for fifteen minutes gives you the needed drive to begin. If you decide to end it at the end of that time, you will probably feel great because you got something done.

However, you may choose to continue since you are already out and make it a half hour journey. Whichever way you go, you have already succeeded.

Get your motivation revived!

Never underestimate the rewards of little exercises. Even a little bike ride or a five minutes' walk could help in lightening you up and boosting your energy. Despite the fact that its rewards may not necessarily compare with that of longer workout sessions, the fifteen-minute plan may just be the secret to driving you back to the much needed regular exercise plan.

Maintain it for three days

It is scientific fact that a body which is at rest remains at rest, however, the moment it begins to move, then momentum will be picked up and it keeps on moving. When you begin an exercise plan or a dietary program, you will need to overcome your inertia and you will then have to increase your momentum. On a general note, if you engage in an activity minimum three days at a stretch, you should be able to get back on the right track.

Hence, ensure that you do anything necessary to begin and then maintain it for about three whole days. By this time, you will have developed the needed rhythm which should get you going.

Conclusion

Thank you again for downloading this book!

I hope this book was able to help you to get your motivation re-ignited to lose weight and keep fit.

The next step is to act upon the content options and your life will never be the same again!

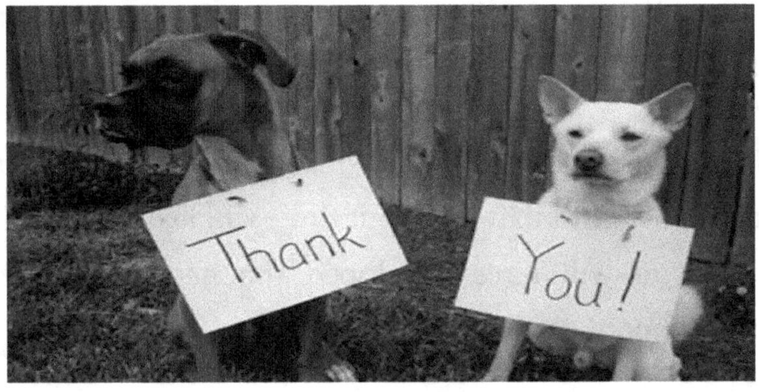

Finally, if you enjoyed this book, then I'd like to ask you for a favor, would you be kind enough to leave a review for this book on Amazon? It'd be greatly appreciated!

Click here to leave a review for this book on Amazon!

Thank you and good luck!